Ketogenic Instant Pot Cookbook

Low Carb Recipes for Your Pressure Cooker, Easy Recipes for Healthy Eating to Lose Weight Fast

OLIVIA STRATTON

Table of Contents

Ketogenic Diet Tips

A keto diet has proved to be very effective. It is a popular low carb diet that makes your liver produce ketones to be used as energy for your body. The ketogenic diet also causes blood sugar and insulin levels reductions.

1. You need to stay hydrated all the time

Specialists recommend drinking 30 oz of water in the first hour once you wake up and add another 30-46 oz of water before noon time. In order to stay properly hydrated you should be drinking at least 100-120 ounces of water on a daily basis.

2. Exercise regularly

Regular resistance training exercises along with running and low-intensity exercise help to balance the level of sugar in blood and improve the ability to get into and maintain ketosis.

3. Practice intermittent fasting

If you want to get yourself into ketosis and maintain it, intermittent fasting will be the best option for you, as with intermittent fasting you will reduce calories and stop consummation of protein or carbs. However, it is strongly recommended to start consuming low quantities of carbs for at least couple of days before starting intermittent fasting as not to get a hypoglycemic episode.

4. Wisely choose carbs that you consume

Ketogenic diet is a low-carb diet and it is recommended to consume nutrient rich carbohydrate sources such as non-starchy veggies and small amounts of low-glycemic fruits.

5. Use MCT oil wherever you can

Consumption of high quality medium chain triglyceride (MCT) oil will allow you to consume more protein/carbs and maintain ketosis. Doing this is probably the best thing you can do to actually get into ketosis and maintain it.

6. Keep stress as low as possible

Stress shuts down the ability to maintain the ketosis. If you are stressing a lot, maybe you should reset your goal to simply stay on a lower carb, anti-inflammatory diet for some time.

7. Get enough sleep

If you do not get enough sleep or the quality of your sleep is poor, you will not be able to get into and maintain the ketosis. Thus, make sure you do sleep well and enough.

Instant Pot Useful Tips

1. Start with carefully reading the instructions for your device

Every pressure cooker comes with a manual that you should carefully study, as it contains terms of use, additional useful tips, and, most importantly, information on how use it safely.

2. Store it right

After finishing your cooking, wash the cooker and put it into storage. Make sure to check the valves and clean those as well.

3. Do not forget to add liquid

Pressure cooker needs liquid to build up steam pressure inside to actually cook the food. This means you need to make sure to add liquid to the ingredients.

4. Do not overfill the cooker

All modern pressure cookers have minimum and maximum marks on the inside of the cooking pot. Make sure not to exceed those. When cooking with liquid make sure to avoid filling more than half full, as filling more that can lead to spill.

5. Right heat

You should make sure to choose the right heat for cooking, as it is one of the key elements for successful cooking in the pressure cooker. Check the needed recipe for more details.

6. Right timing

You should make sure to choose the right timing for cooking, as it is one of the key elements for successful cooking in the pressure cooker. Check the needed recipe for more details.

7. Brown the ingredients

Ingredients in the pressure cooker do not brown, so make sure to actually brown those before you start cooking. If you have a modern electric pressure cooker you can do that in it as well.

8. Slice the ingredients to the right size

Slice food into even pieces for even cooking. Larger slices will cook slower, smaller slices faster. Check the needed recipe for more details.

9. Release the pressure

There are usually two ways to release steam in your pressure cooker: a) turning a pressure release valve – use oven gloves for this as hot steam will rush out, and c) or open the top lid. However, make sure to carefully open the top lid as not to get burnt.

Soft Keto Chicken

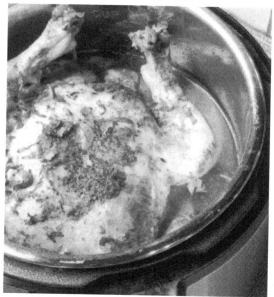

Cooking Time: 30 minutes

Servings: 10

Ingredients

    4 pound (1 whole) organic chicken

    1 teaspoon paprika

    1 tablespoon coconut oil

    1 teaspoon thyme, dried

    1½ cups chicken bone broth

    2 tablespoons lemon juice

    ¼ teaspoon freshly ground black pepper

    6 garlic cloves, peeled

    ½ teaspoon sea salt

Instructions

1. Mix pepper, salt, thyme, and paprika in a mixing bowl.
2. Season the chicken with the mixture.
3. Put coconut oil into Instant Pot.
4. Press "Sauté" button and put seasoned chicken breast side down into Instant Pot.
5. Sauté chicken for 6-7 minutes with the lid open.
6. Turn the chicken over, add garlic cloves, lemon juice, and broth.
7. Close the lid, and turn the vent to "Sealed".
8. Press "Manual" button, set the timer for 25 minutes and set "Pressure" to high.
9. Once the timer is up, press "Cancel" button and allow the pressure to be released naturally, until the float valve drops down. Open the lid.

NOTE: Make sure the pressure is fully released before opening the lid, so you do not get burnt.

10. Set it aside to cool for 5 minutes before you can carve the chicken.

Nutritional info

Calories: 311

Fats (g): 7.7

Net carbs (g): 1.4

Protein (g): 25.4

Chicken Tikka Masala

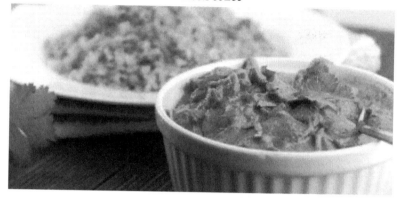

Cooking Time: 20 minutes

Servings: 4

Chicken & Marinade Ingredients

  1 pound chicken breasts, boneless, skinless and chopped into small bite-sized pieces

  1 tablespoon garam masala

  1 cup (7 oz.) plain 2% fat Greek yogurt

  1 teaspoon black pepper

  1 tablespoon lemon juice (Approx. 1/2 lemon)

  1/4 teaspoon ground ginger

Sauce Ingredients

  0.5 cup tomato puree or sauce

  4 teaspoons garam masala

  5 garlic cloves, minced

  1/2 teaspoon turmeric

  1/2 teaspoon paprika

  1/4 teaspoon cayenne

  1/2 teaspoon salt

1 cup heavy whipping cream (added last)

cilantro, freshly chopped

Instructions

1. Mix all marinade ingredients (except chicken meat) in a mixing bowl.
2. Add chicken to the marinade and stir until evenly mixed.
3. Refrigerate chicken in marinade for at least 1 hour.
4. Press "Sauté" button, set "Temperature" to medium.
5. Put chicken in marinade into Instant Pot.
6. Sauté and stir chicken in marinade with the lid open until evenly cooked.
7. Put all sauce ingredients (except the whipping cream) over the sautéed chicken, and stir until evenly mixed.
8. Close the lid, and turn the vent to "Sealed".
9. Press "Manual" button, set the timer for 10 minutes and set "Pressure" to high.
10. Once the timer is up press "Cancel" button and turn the steam release handle to "Venting" position for quick release, until the float valve drops down.
11. Press "Sauté" button, set "Temperature" to low.
12. Put whipping cream into Instant Pot once it warms up.
13. Stir well and simmer until the sauce reaches your desired thickness.
14. Serve garnished with cilantro.

Nutritional info

Calories: 537

Fats (g): 22.8

Net carbs (g): 5.8

Protein (g): 56.9

Parm Spaghetti Squash with Chicken

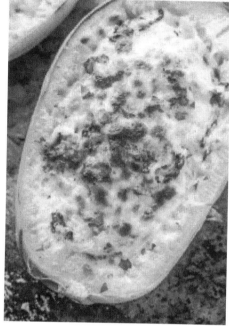

Cooking Time: 22 minutes

Servings: 2-3

Ingredients

  1 spaghetti squash, split in half and seeded

  1 pound chicken, cooked and chopped into cubes

  0.5 cup marinara sauce

  1 cup water

  7 oz mozzarella cheese

Instructions

1.   Pour water into Instant Pot.

2. Place the trivet into Instant Pot.
3. Put squash halves on the trivet.
4. Close the lid, and turn the vent to "Sealed".
5. Press "Manual" button, set the timer for 20 minutes and set "Pressure" to high.
6. Once the timer is up press "Cancel" button and turn the steam release handle to "Venting" position for quick release, until the float valve drops down.
7. Open the lid.

NOTE: Make sure the pressure is fully released before opening the lid, so you do not get burnt.

8. Take out spaghetti squash and shred with a fork.
9. Pour marinara sauce over spaghetti squash and stir until evenly mixed.
10. Put chicken cubes over spaghetti squash.
11. Top with mozzarella cheese.

Nutritional info

Calories: 300

Fats (g): 5.3

Net carbs (g): 4

Protein (g): 34

Spicy Creamy Chicken Breasts

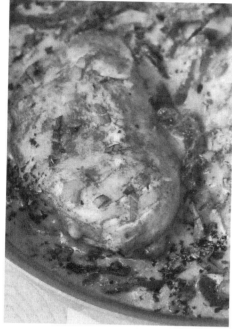

Cooking Time: 12 minutes

Servings: 2-4

Ingredients

    1 pound chicken breast, boneless

    3 jalapenos, sliced

    8 oz cream cheese

    ¾ cup sour cream

    8 oz cheddar cheese

    ½ cup water

Instructions

1. Put water, cream cheese, sliced jalapenos and chicken breast into Instant Pot.
2. Close the lid, and turn the vent to "Sealed".
3. Press "Manual" button, set the timer for 12 minutes and set "Pressure" to high.
4. Once the timer is up press "Cancel" button and turn the steam release handle to "Venting" position for quick release, until the float valve drops down.
5. Open the lid.

NOTE: Make sure the pressure is fully released before opening the lid, so you do not get burnt.

6. Put sour cream and cheddar cheese into Instant Pot and stir until evenly mixed.

Nutritional info

Calories: 650

Fats (g): 50

Net carbs (g): 4.7

Protein (g): 43

Crack Chicken

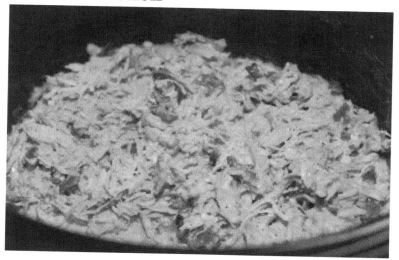

Cooking Time: 25 minutes

Servings: 6-8

Ingredients

6-8 bacon slices

1 teaspoon ranch seasoning

2 pounds chicken breast, boneless

1 cup water

8 oz cream cheese

4 oz cheddar cheese

3 tablespoons corn starch

Instructions

1. Put cream cheese and chicken breast into Instant Pot.
2. Season chicken with ranch seasoning, pour water into Instant Pot.

3. Close the lid, and turn the vent to "Sealed".
4. Press "Manual" button, set the timer for 25 minutes and set "Pressure" to high.
5. Once the timer is up press "Cancel" button and turn the steam release handle to "Venting" position for quick release, until the float valve drops down.
6. Open the lid.

NOTE: Make sure the pressure is fully released before opening the lid, so you do not get burnt.

7. Take out chicken and shred it with a fork.
8. Set "Temperature" on low and put whisk cornstarch into Instant Pot.
9. Add shredded chicken and cheddar cheese and stir until evenly mixed.
10. Add the bacon slices and stir.

Nutritional info

Calories: 359

Fats (g): 21.9

Net carbs (g): 4.3

Protein (g): 33.5

Chicken Breasts Keto

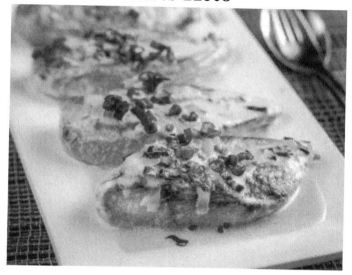

Cooking Time: 12 minutes

Servings: 4-6

Ingredients

4 chicken breasts, frozen

1 cup chicken broth (or 1 cup water and 1 teaspoon chicken bouillon)

1 cup water

1/2 teaspoon salt

Instructions

1. Put chicken breasts into Instant Pot, add water and salt.
2. Close the lid, and turn the vent to "Sealed".
3. Press "Poultry" button, set the timer for 12 minutes and set "Pressure" to high.

4. Once the timer is up, press "Cancel" button and allow the pressure to be released naturally, until the float valve drops down.
5. Turn the steam release handle to "Venting" position for quick release, until the float valve drops down.

NOTE: Make sure the pressure is fully released before opening the lid, so you do not get burnt.

6. Shred chicken and store with chicken broth in a refrigerator.

Nutritional info

Calories: 326

Fats (g): 12

Net carbs (g): 0.2

Protein (g): 40.1

Bone Broth

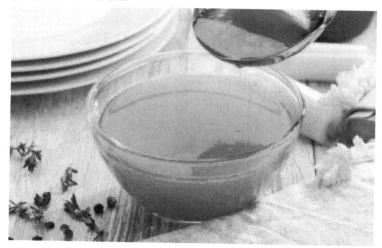

Cooking Time: 60 minutes

Servings: 12

Ingredients

1 chicken carcass, cooked, with most meat drippings removed

1 small onion, skin on & quartered

1" ginger knob

2 garlic cloves

1 cup celery tops, chopped

3.5-4 quarts water, filtered

2 tablespoons apple cider vinegar

Instructions

1. Put every solid ingredient into Instant Pot.
2. Pour water up to the 4 quarts mark.
3. Stir to mix.

4. Close the lid of the instant pot, and set vent to "Sealed".
5. Press "Manual" button, set the timer for 60 minutes and set "Pressure" to high.
6. Once the timer is up press "Cancel" button and turn the steam release handle to "Venting" position for quick release, until the float valve drops down.
7. Open the lid.

NOTE: Make sure the pressure is fully released before opening the lid, so you do not get burnt.

8. Set broth aside to cool for 60 minutes before taking out the solids.
9. Put broth into container and season with sea salt.
10. Refrigerate for up to 8 hours or overnight.
11. Remove fat from the broth's top.

Nutritional info

Calories: 260

Fats (g): 10

Net carbs (g): 2

Protein (g): 15

Spaghetti Squash Chicken Marsala

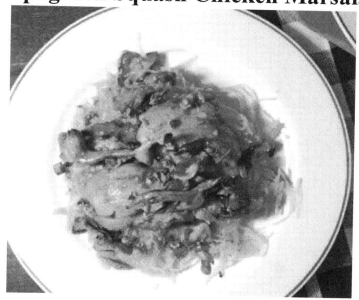

Cooking Time: 28 minutes

Servings: 4-6

Ingredients

2 pounds chicken thighs or breast, boneless
2 garlic cloves, minced
1 teaspoon coconut oil
1 cup Marsala Cooking wine
1 cup shitake mushrooms, sliced
1 cup water
3 tablespoons Xanthan Gum
½ cup organic chicken broth
large spaghetti squash
fresh basil

salt, black pepper, to taste

Instructions

1. Place the steam rack into Instant Pot.
2. Put spaghetti squash on the steam rack and pour water.
3. Close the lid, and turn the vent to "Sealed".
4. Press "Manual" button, set the timer for 20 minutes and set "Pressure" to high.
5. Once the timer is up, press "Cancel" button and allow the pressure to be released naturally, until the float valve drops down.
6. Open the lid.

NOTE: Make sure the pressure is fully released before opening the lid, so you do not get burnt.

7. Take squash out, set aside, pour water out and dry Instant Pot.
8. Put coconut oil into Instant Pot and press "Sauté" button.
9. Put chicken, pepper and salt into Instant Pot and brown the chicken.
10. Put Marsala wine, mushrooms and garlic over the browned chicken.
11. Close the lid, and turn the vent to "Sealed".
12. Press "Manual" button, set the timer for 8 minutes and set "Pressure" to high.
13. Once the timer is up press "Cancel" button and turn the steam release handle to "Venting" position for quick release, until the float valve drops down.
14. Open the lid.
15. Put chicken broth into Instant Pot and stir until evenly mixed.
16. Take 1/4 cup cooking juice out of Instant Pot and put into a mixing bowl.
17. Mix 1/4 cup cooking juice with gelatin until gelatin dissolves.

18. Put the gelatin mixture into Instant Pot.
19. Slice spaghetti squash into two and get rid of squash seeds.
20. Peel off squash rind with a fork.
21. Top with Marsala sauce, mushrooms, chicken and garnish with fresh basil.

Nutritional info

Calories: 400

Fats (g): 15.6

Net carbs (g): 4.8

Protein (g): 26.3

Smoked Sausage Stew & Chicken

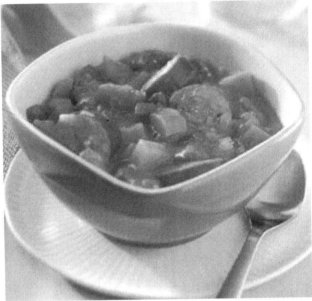

Cooking Time: 30 minutes

Servings: 6

Ingredients

    1 pound chicken thighs, boneless, skinless

    1 tablespoon coconut oil

    1 pound andouille pork sausage

    1 medium white onion, thinly sliced

    1 medium tomato, chopped

    1 bell pepper, diced

    2 celery stalks, chopped

    2 cups water or bone broth

    1 large carrot, chopped

    6 garlic cloves, minced

1/4 cup parsley, minced

1 teaspoon thyme

1 teaspoon salt

1/2 teaspoon red chili flakes, crushed

1/2 teaspoon smoked paprika

1/4 teaspoon cayenne

1/4 teaspoon black pepper

hot sauce (if desired)

1 bay leaf

Instructions

1. Put coconut oil into Instant Pot.
2. Press "Sauté" button, put sausage and chicken into Instant Pot.
3. Sauté till the meat is evenly cooked.
4. Take out cooked meat and set aside.
5. Put celery, onions, bell peppers, and carrots into Instant Pot.
6. Press "Sauté" button and stir from time to time.
7. Put minced garlic into Instant Pot and continue sautéing.
8. Put chopped tomatoes and broth into Instant Pot.
9. Continue sautéing until simmering.
10. Once cooled, slice sausage and chicken into small chunks.
11. Put sausage, chicken, spices and the minced parsley into Instant Pot, stir until evenly mixed.
12. Close the lid, and turn the vent to "Sealed".
13. Press "Soup" button, set the timer for 5-10 minutes and set "Pressure" to high.
14. Once the timer is up press "Cancel" button and turn the steam release handle to "Venting" position for quick release, until the float valve drops down.
15. Open the lid.

NOTE: Make sure the pressure is fully released before opening the lid, so you do not get burnt.

16. Serve warm, topped with hot sauce (if desired).

Nutritional info

Calories: 331

Fats (g): 37.3

Net carbs (g): 6.5

Protein (g): 25.6

Frozen Chicken Breasts

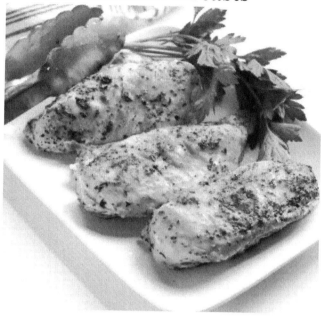

Cooking Time: 12 minutes

Servings: 6

Ingredients

4 chicken breasts, frozen

1 cup chicken broth (or 1 cup water and 1 teaspoon chicken bouillon)

1 cup water

1/2 teaspoon salt

Instructions

1. Put chicken breasts into Instant Pot, add water and salt.
2. Close the lid, and turn the vent to "Sealed".

3. Press "Manual" button, set the timer for 25 minutes and set "Pressure" to medium.
4. Once the timer is up, press "Cancel" button and allow the pressure to be released naturally, until the float valve drops down.
5. Turn the steam release handle to "Venting" position for quick release, until the float valve drops down.
6. Open the lid.

NOTE: Make sure the pressure is fully released before opening the lid, so you do not get burnt.

7. Shred chicken and store with chicken broth in a refrigerator.

Nutritional info

Calories: 513

Fats (g): 26.9

Net carbs (g): 0.2

Protein (g): 22.2

Chicken & Broth

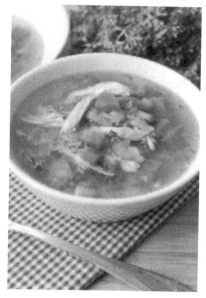

Cooking Time: 40 minutes

Servings: 4

Ingredients

    2 carrots, peeled & sliced

    2 tablespoons cooking oil

    1 yellow or white onion, sliced or chopped

    2 celery stalks, sliced

    2 teaspoons salt

    4 pounds chicken

    2 bay leaves

    1 tablespoons black peppercorns

    8-12 cups water

    fresh herbs

    garlic cloves

Instructions

1. Put cooking oil into Instant Pot.
2. Press "Sauté" button and put onions, celery and carrots into Instant Pot and sauté for 3-5 minutes.
3. Put the chicken breast side down over veggies into Instant Pot.
4. Add bay leaves, peppercorns and salt.
5. Pour sufficient amount water into Instant Pot until the chicken is just covered.
6. Close the lid, and turn the vent to "Sealed".
7. Press "Manual" button, set the timer for 40 minutes and set "Pressure" to high.
8. Once the timer is up, press "Cancel" button and allow the pressure to be released naturally, until the float valve drops down.
9. Open the lid.

NOTE: Make sure the pressure is fully released before opening the lid, so you do not get burnt.

10. Take out the chicken, debone the meat.
11. Strain and degrease the broth.
12. Serve chicken with a little broth and refrigerate the left over broth.

Nutritional info

Calories: 476

Fats (g): 22.7

Net carbs (g): 6

Protein (g): 32.2

Chicken Cacciatore

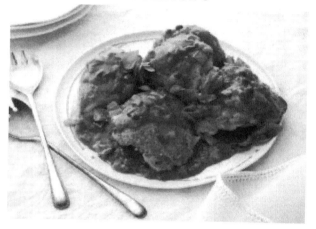

Cooking Time: 15 minutes

Servings: 6

Ingredients

3 shallots, chopped
1-2 tablespoon olive oil
1 green bell pepper, seeded & diced
4 garlic cloves, crushed
1 package (8-10 oz) sliced mushrooms
1/2 cup organic veggie or chicken broth
2 cans organic tomatoes, crushed
5-6 chicken breasts, boneless skinless
1 can black olives, pitted
2 tablespoons organic tomato paste
1/2 teaspoon or more red pepper
fresh parsley
sea salt
black pepper

Instructions

1. Put olive oil into Instant Pot.
2. Press "Sauté" button, put bell pepper and shallots into Instant Pot.
3. Sauté and stir for 2 minutes (approx), until the shallot is slightly tenderized.
4. Pour broth into Instant Pot and boil it for 2-3 minutes.
5. Put garlic and mushrooms into Instant Pot, then put chicken on top of the veggies.
6. Top with crushed tomatoes and make sure NOT to stir, and then top with tomato paste.
7. Close the lid, and turn the vent to "Sealed".
8. Press "Manual" button, set the timer for 8 minutes and set "Pressure" to high.
9. Once the timer is up, press "Cancel" button and allow the pressure to be released naturally, until the float valve drops down.
10. Open the lid.

NOTE: Make sure the pressure is fully released before opening the lid, so you do not get burnt.

11. Add pepper, salt, red pepper flakes and olives.
12. Stir until evenly mixed and serve over cabbage or alone.

Nutritional info

Calories: 320

Fats (g): 30

Net carbs (g): 5

Protein (g): 39.7

Garlic Lemon Chicken

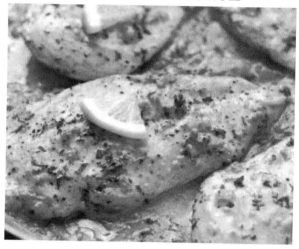

Cooking Time: 25 minutes

Servings: 2-4

Ingredients

> 1-2 pounds chicken thighs or breasts
> 1 onion, diced
> 1 teaspoon sea salt
> 5 garlic cloves, minced
> 1 tablespoon ghee, lard or avocado oil
> 1 teaspoon parsley, dried
> 1/2 cup homemade chicken broth
> 1/4 cup white cooking wine
> 1/4 teaspoon paprika
> 3-4 teaspoon (or additional) arrowroot flour
> 1 large lemon juiced (or more if needed)

Instructions

1. Put cooking fat and diced onions into Instant Pot.

2. Press "Sauté" button and sauté onions for 5-10 minutes until softened and translucent.
3. Put every other ingredient (excluding the arrowroot flour) into Instant Pot.
4. Close the lid, and turn the vent to "Sealed".
5. Press "Manual" button, set the timer for 12 minutes and set "Pressure" to high.
6. Once the timer is up press "Cancel" button and turn the steam release handle to "Venting" position for quick release, until the float valve drops down.
7. Open the lid.

NOTE: Make sure the pressure is fully released before opening the lid, so you do not get burnt.

8. Take 1/4 cup cooking juice out of Instant Pot and mix arrow root flour in mixing bowl.
9. Put the mixture back into Instant Pot and stir until evenly mixed.

Nutritional info

Calories: 255

Fats (g): 29.1

Net carbs (g): 4.8

Protein (g): 34.1

Hungarian Chicken

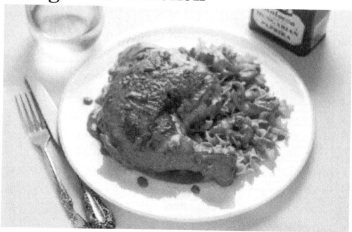

Cooking Time: 30 minutes

Servings: 4

Ingredients

1 tablespoon vegetable oil

3 1/2-4 pounds chicken leg quarters, bone-in and skin removed

1 small onion, well diced

1 teaspoon salt

zucchini noodles, cooked

1/2 cup chicken broth

2 teaspoons hot paprika

1/2 cup sour cream

1 medium tomato, skin removed & coarsely chopped

Instructions

1. Put vegetable oil into Instant Pot.

2. Press "Sauté" button, add chicken and brown it for 4-5 minutes until golden brown.
3. Take out chicken from Instant Pot.
4. Put broth, onions, paprika, and browned chicken back into Instant Pot.
5. Put tomatoes on top of chicken, and sprinkle it with salt. Make sure NOT to stir.
6. Close the lid, and turn the vent to "Sealed".
7. Press "Manual" button, set the timer for 10 minutes and set "Pressure" to high.
8. Once the timer is up, press "Cancel" button and allow the pressure to be released naturally, until the float valve drops down.
9. Open the lid.
10. Take out chicken from Instant Pot and let it cool.
11. Press "Sauté" button, and sauté for 15 minutes until the leftover liquid thickens.
12. Whisk sour cream in a mixing bowl until it is of a fine consistency.
13. Take 1/4 cup cooking juice out of Instant Pot and add to the sour cream mixture and stir until evenly mixed.
14. Put cream mixture and chicken back into Instant Pot and simmer for few minutes.
15. Serve zucchini noodles with chicken topped with a small amount of sauce.

Nutritional info

Calories: 260

Fats (g): 19

Net carbs (g): 5.9

Protein (g): 16.3

Zuppa Toscana

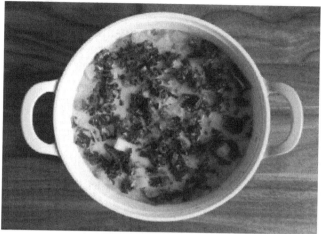

Cooking Time: 20 minutes

Servings: 6

Ingredients

 2 tablespoons avocado or olive oil
 3 garlic cloves, minced
 1 medium sized yellow onion, chopped
 1 cauliflower head, separated into florets
 1 pound Italian Sausage, chicken or turkey
 2 teaspoons basil, dried
 5 cups chicken broth
 2 cups fresh kale, chopped
 1 teaspoon fennel, dried
 1 tablespoon red pepper, crushed
 ½ cup heavy cream or full fat coconut milk
 salt, pepper, to taste

Instructions

1. Put avocado oil or olive oil into Instant Pot.
2. Press "Sauté" button, put chopped onions into Instant Pot and sauté for 2-3 minutes until softened.
3. Add sausage and garlic and brown for 5 minutes.
4. Press "Cancel" button, add broth into the instant pot, and stir until incorporate.
5. Add herbs and cauliflower florets.
6. Close the lid, and turn the vent to "Sealed".
7. Press "Manual" button, set the timer for 12 minutes and set "Pressure" to high.
8. Once the timer is up press "Cancel" button and turn the steam release handle to "Venting" position for quick release, until the float valve drops down.
9. Open the lid.

NOTE: Make sure the pressure is fully released before opening the lid, so you do not get burnt.

10. Press "Sauté" button, pit kale into the instant pot, and sauté kale until it is wilted.
11. Add heavy cream or coconut milk, stir until evenly mixed, and then sprinkle with pepper, salt, and crushed red pepper

Nutritional info

Calories: 410

Fats (g): 30

Net carbs (g): 6

Protein (g): 22

Pumpkin Turkey Chili

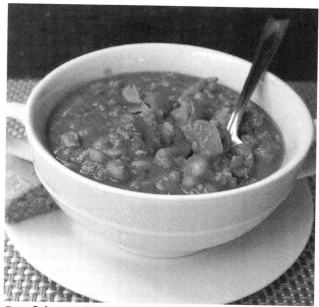

Cooking Time: 20 minutes

Servings: 6

Ingredients

  1 tablespoon coconut oil

  1 garlic clove, minced

  1 pound ground turkey

  1 (14.5 ounce) can diced tomatoes

  2 cups pumpkin puree

  1 1/2 tablespoons chili powder

  ¼ teaspoon oregano

  ¼ teaspoon cumin

  1/2 cup shredded Cheddar cheese

  1/2 cup sour cream

1/2 teaspoon ground black pepper

1 dash salt

1 cup water

Instructions

1. Pour oil to the pressure cooker. Press "Sauté" button, set "Temperature" to medium.
2. Heat the oil in until shimmering. Add ground turkey and brown a bit.
3. Add garlic, onion and pumpkin, mix well.
4. Sprinkle with chili powder, salt, oregano, cumin and mix again to coat the pumpkin evenly.
5. Add water and close the Instant Pot lid.
6. Press "Manual" button, set the timer for 20 minutes and set "Pressure" to high.
7. Once the timer is up press "Cancel" button and turn the steam release handle to "Venting" position for quick release, until the float valve drops down.
8. Serve topped with Cheddar cheese.

Nutritional info

Calories: 330

Fats (g): 20

Net carbs (g): 8

Protein (g): 15

Turkey Tetrazzini with Zucchini Pasta

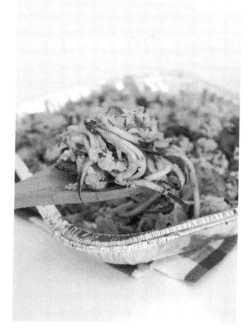

Cooking Time: 25 minutes

Servings: 8

Ingredients

2 large zucchini, peeled into noodle ribbons

2 tablespoons olive oil

½ lemon zest

1/3 lemon juice

1/2 cup unsalted butter

2 cups fresh mushrooms, sliced

1 cup onion, minced

2 stalks celery, diced

16 oz vegetable or chicken stock

1/2 cup sour cream

1 teaspoon salt

1/4 teaspoon ground black pepper

¼ teaspoon dried thyme

4 cups cooked turkey breast, chopped

1 cup grated Parmesan cheese

paprika to taste

Instructions

1. Press "Sauté" button on your Instant Pot, set "Temperature" to medium. Heat up for 1-2 minutes.
2. Add olive oil, lemon zest and salt, stir for 20-30 seconds.
3. Add zucchini noodles and lemon juice, stir for 30 more seconds and turn off the Pot. Sprinkle with ½ cup Parmesan cheese and set aside.
4. Add butter to the Instant Pot, press "Sauté" button on your Instant Pot, set "Temperature" to medium.
5. Add celery, onion and mushrooms, sauté for 4-5 minutes.
6. Add turkey, thyme and broth to the Instant Pot. Close the lid, and turn the vent to "Sealed".
7. Press "Manual" button, set the timer for 9 minutes and set "Pressure" to high.
8. Once the timer is up press "Cancel" button and turn the steam release handle to "Venting" position for quick release, until the float valve drops down.
9. Stir in the rest of Parmesan cheese, add salt and sour cream. Stir for 1-2 minutes until the sauce thickens.
10. Serve on zucchini noodles.

Nutritional info

Calories: 320

Fats (g): 25

Net carbs (g): 6.2

Protein (g): 12

Apple Turkey Curry

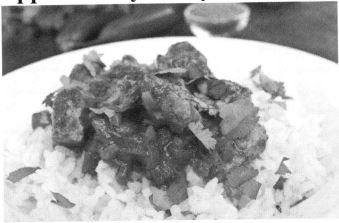

Cooking Time: 20 minutes

Servings: 3

Ingredients

2 tablespoons olive oil

1 cup onion, sliced

2 tablespoons lemon juice

1/2 pound cooked turkey breasts, chopped

1 apple, cored and finely sliced

1/2 cup full fat yogurt

1 teaspoon Curry powder

1 cup water

Instructions

1. Press "Sauté" button on your Instant Pot, set "Temperature" to medium. Heat up for 1-2 minutes.
2. Add oil and onion, sauté until golden brown. Add garlic, sauté for 20 more seconds. Add Curry powder.

3. Add apple, turkey, water, salt and pepper. Mix well.
4. Close the lid, and turn the vent to "Sealed".
5. Press "Manual" button, set the timer for 12 minutes and set "Pressure" to high.
6. Once the timer is up press "Cancel" button and turn the steam release handle to "Venting" position for quick release, until the float valve drops down.
7. Open the lid. Add yogurt, sprinkle with lemon juice and mix well.
8. Press "Sauté" button and cook for 5 minutes stirring well.

Nutritional info

Calories: 320

Fats (g): 28

Net carbs (g): 5

Protein (g): 18

Turkey Tenderloin

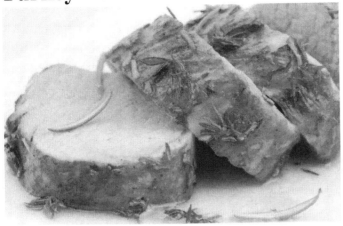

Cooking Time: 20 minutes

Servings: 4

Ingredients

- 1/3 cup chicken broth
- 1 pound turkey tenderloin
- 3 tablespoons soy sauce
- 1 tablespoon Dijon-style prepared mustard
- 2 teaspoons dried rosemary, crushed

Instructions

1. Mix soy sauce, mustard and rosemary in a small bowl.
2. Put turkey tenderloin into the Instant Pot, add the soy sauce mixture and chicken broth.
3. Close the lid, and turn the vent to "Sealed".
4. Press "Poultry" button, set the timer for 18 minutes and set "Pressure" to high.

5. Once the timer is up, press "Cancel" button and allow the pressure to be released naturally, until the float valve drops down. Open the lid.

NOTE: Make sure the pressure is fully released before opening the lid, so you do not get burnt.

Nutritional info

Calories: 134

Fats (g): 29

Net carbs (g): 2.4

Protein (g): 19.5

Turkey Posole

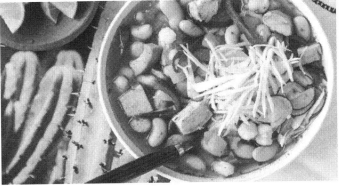

Cooking Time: 10 minutes

Servings: 8

Ingredients

3 tablespoons olive oil

1 yellow onion, cubed

2 garlic cloves, minced

4 cups turkey soup

4 cups cooked turkey, cubed

1 (4 ounce) can green chili peppers, chopped

1 can white hominy, drained

1 tablespoon chili powder

2 tablespoons cumin

2 tablespoons dried oregano

1 cup water

salt and pepper, to taste

Instructions

1. Add oil to the Instant Pot, press "Sauté" button, set "Temperature" to medium.
2. Add cooked turkey, garlic, onion, salt, pepper, oregano, chili powder and paprika.
3. Sauté till turkey is browned, for about 10 minutes.
4. Add cumin, green chili peppers and water, mix to blend.
5. Close the lid, and turn the vent to "Sealed".
6. Press "Manual" button, set the timer for 15 minutes and set "Pressure" to high.
7. Once the timer is up, press "Cancel" button and allow the pressure to be released naturally, until the float valve drops down. Open the lid.

NOTE: Make sure the pressure is fully released before opening the lid, so you do not get burnt.

8. Once the pressure is released, open the lid and add hominy. Mix well.

Nutritional info

Calories: 260

Fats (g): 20

Net carbs (g): 4

Protein (g): 16

Braised Beef Short Keto Ribs

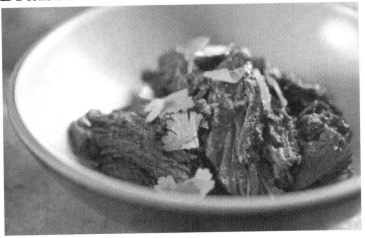

Cooking Time: 35 minutes

Servings: 4

Ingredients

4 pounds beef short ribs

1 tablespoon vegetable oil/ avocado oil/bacon fat or beef fat

3 garlic cloves

1 onion, skin on and quartered

water

kosher salt

Instructions

1. Sprinkle salt over ribs.
2. Add oil into Instant Pot.
3. Press "Sauté" button, add ribs into Instant Pot.

4. Sear ribs until browned, then add garlic, onion and pour water 2 inches of water into Instant Pot.
5. Close the lid, and turn the vent to "Sealed".
6. Press "Manual" button, set the timer for 35 minutes and set "Pressure" to high.
7. Once the timer is up press "Cancel" button and turn the steam release handle to "Venting" position for quick release, until the float valve drops down.
8. Open the lid.

NOTE: Make sure the pressure is fully released before opening the lid, so you do not get burnt.

9. Take the ribs out, and debone the meat, then strain the cooking juices and get rid of the fat residue on the top.
10. Store left-over broth in a refrigerator.

Nutritional info

Calories: 454

Fats (g): 40.9

Net carbs (g): 3.3

Protein (g): 31.4

Beef Short Ribs & Bacon

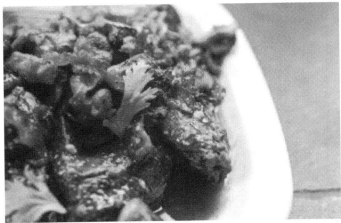

Cooking Time: 45 minutes

Servings: 4

Ingredients

  4 pounds (approx) beef short ribs, large

  2 bacon slices, chopped

  2 tablespoon, vegetable oil

  3 garlic cloves, minced or pressed

  1 large onion, chopped

  1 cup beef both

  1/2 cup dry red wine

  1 tablespoon cornstarch

  2 tablespoons tomato paste

  1 tablespoon water

Instructions

1. Sprinkle pepper and salt over ribs.
2. Put cooking oil into Instant Pot, and press "Sauté" button.

3. Sear ribs until browned, then take browned ribs out of Instant Pot.
4. Put bacon slices into Instant Pot and sear until crisp and brown.
5. Add chopped onions and cook for 3 minutes until soft.
6. Add garlic and cook for 1 additional minute until fragrant.
7. Pour wine into Instant Pot, add ribs with tomato paste and beef broth.
8. Close the lid, and turn the vent to "Sealed".
9. Press "Manual" button, set the timer for 40 minutes and set "Pressure" to high.
10. Once the timer is up press "Cancel" button and turn the steam release handle to "Venting" position for quick release, until the float valve drops down.
11. Open the lid.
12. Take ribs out, strain cooking grease, then put cooking juices back into Instant Pot.
13. Mix water, cornstarch and whisk in a mixing bowl.
14. Put the mixture into Instant Pot over cooking juices.
15. Press "Sauté" button and sauté cooking juices until thickened.
16. Put ribs into Instant Pot, and stir until evenly mixed.
17. Cover instant pot and let sit for 10 minutes to warm ribs.
18. Serve over zucchini noodles.

Nutritional info

Calories: 533

Fats (g): 45.2

Net carbs (g): 5.3

Protein (g): 36.6

Noodle-less lasagna

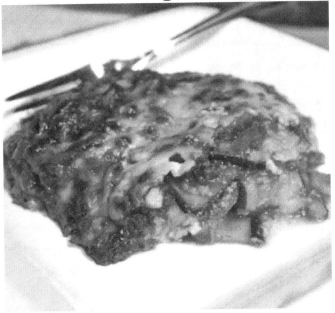

Cooking Time: 25 minutes

Servings: 8

Ingredients

1 pound ground beef

1 onion, small

2 garlic cloves, minced

1/2 cup Parmesan cheese

1 1/2 cups Ricotta cheese

1 jar (25 oz.) marinara sauce

1 egg, large

8 oz Mozzarella, sliced

Instructions

1. Add onion, garlic, and ground beef into Instant Pot.
2. Press "Sauté" button and brown the ground beef.
3. Mix egg, Parmesan and Ricotta cheese in a mixing bowl.
4. Pour marinara sauce into Instant Pot, take out half of beef mixture and set aside.
5. Add 1/2 (4 oz.) Mozzarella to the beef sauce, then add 1/2 Ricotta cheese on top of the mozzarella cheese layer, and put beef sauce back into Instant Pot.
6. Add some of the remaining Mozzarella over the meat sauce, saving some cheese for later, and then put the other half of Ricotta cheese into Instant Pot.
7. Close the lid, and turn the vent to "Sealed".
8. Press "Manual" button, set the timer for 8-10 minutes and set "Pressure" to high.
9. Once the timer is up, press "Cancel" button and allow the pressure to be released naturally, until the float valve drops down.
10. Open the lid.

NOTE: Make sure the pressure is fully released before opening the lid, so you do not get burnt.

11. Add Parmesan cheese over lasagna and top with remaining Mozzarella.
12. Close the lid and allow cheese to melt.

Nutritional info

Calories: 311

Fats (g): 25.4

Net carbs (g): 7.5

Protein (g): 35

Creamy Sauce & Meatballs

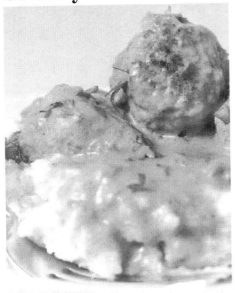

Cooking Time: 10 minutes

Servings: 5

Ingredients

    1 ½ pound (85/15 or leaner) ground beef

    3 oz parmesan cheese, grated

    2 tablespoons fresh parsley, chopped

    2 eggs

    ½ cup almond flour

    ¼ teaspoon ground black pepper

    1 teaspoon kosher salt

    1 teaspoon onion flakes, dried

    ¼ teaspoon garlic powder

    1/3 cup warm water

    ¼ teaspoons oregano, dried

1 cup marinara sauce

1 teaspoon olive oil

Instructions

1. Mix every ingredient (except olive oil and marinara sauce) into a mixing bowl.
2. Mould the mixture into fifteen (2" each) meatballs.
3. Put olive oil into Instant Pot, then put meatballs and press "Sauté" button to brown meatballs evenly.
4. Put marinara sauce into Instant Pot.
5. Close the lid, and turn the vent to "Sealed".
6. Press "Manual" button, set the timer for 10 minutes and set "Pressure" to low.
7. Once the timer is up press "Cancel" button and turn the steam release handle to "Venting" position for quick release, until the float valve drops down.
8. Open the lid.

NOTE: Make sure the pressure is fully released before opening the lid, so you do not get burnt.

9. Serve spaghetti squash or zucchini noodles topped with sauce and meatballs.

Nutritional info

Calories: 403

Fats (g): 30.5

Net carbs (g): 8.8

Protein (g): 35

Traditional Meatloaf

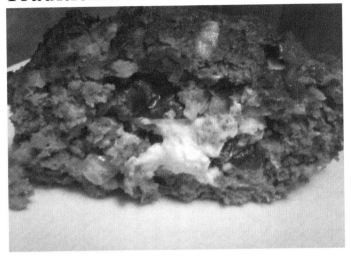

Cooking Time: 30 minutes

Servings: 8

Ingredients

>2 pounds lean ground beef
>
>¼ cup Parmesan cheese, grated
>
>½ cup golden flaxseed meal or almond meal
>
>1 beaten egg, large
>
>¼ cup yellow onion, minced
>
>2 teaspoons Worcestershire sauce
>
>1 tablespoon garlic, minced
>
>1 teaspoon salt
>
>½ teaspoon thyme, dried
>
>1 tablespoon vegetable oil
>
>½ teaspoon pepper
>
>1 tablespoon BBQ sauce or ketchup

1 yellow onion, diced

½ cup beef broth or stock

Instructions

1. Mix salt, pepper, thyme, Worcestershire sauce, garlic, egg, minced onion, cheese, flaxseed meal or almond meal and beef in a mixing bowl.
2. Mould the mixture into a ball shape that will perfectly fit into Instant Pot.
3. Put oil into Instant Pot and press "Sauté" button.
4. Put diced onions into Instant Pot and sauté for 4-5 minutes until the onions are translucent.
5. Add ketchup, beef stock and ball shaped meat loaf.
6. Close the lid, and turn the vent to "Sealed".
7. Press "Manual" button, set the timer for 15 minutes and set "Pressure" to high.
8. Once the timer is up, press "Cancel" button and allow the pressure to be released naturally, until the float valve drops down.
9. Open the lid.

NOTE: Make sure the pressure is fully released before opening the lid, so you do not get burnt.

10. Serve with the left over sauce.

Nutritional info

Calories: 294

Fats (g): 25

Net carbs (g): 3.1

Protein (g): 38.8

Mexi Meatloaf

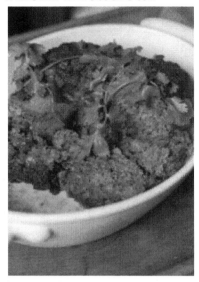

Cooking Time: 40 minutes

Servings: 4

Ingredients

 2 pounds ground grass-fed beef

 1 teaspoon cumin

 1/2 cup + 1/4 cup fire roasted salsa, divided

 1 teaspoon chili powder

 1 teaspoon garlic powder

 1 teaspoon onion powder

 1 teaspoon paprika

 1 teaspoon ground black pepper

 1 teaspoon sea salt

 1 egg, pastured

 1 large yellow onion, diced

1 tablespoon olive oil, avocado oil or ghee

1/4 cup cassava flour or arrowroot or tapioca starch

Instructions

1. Mix every ingredient (except the oil) in a mixing bowl.

NOTE: Leave out 1/4 cup salsa for further use.

2. Mould the mixture into a form of a loaf.
3. Put olive oil, avocado oil or ghee into Instant Pot.
4. Press "Sauté" button, add meatloaf and top with the remaining 1/4 cup salsa.
5. Close the lid, and turn the vent to "Sealed".
6. Press "Meat/Stew" button, set the timer for 35 minutes and set "Pressure" to medium.
7. Once the timer is up press "Cancel" button and turn the steam release handle to "Venting" position for quick release, until the float valve drops down.
8. Open the lid.

NOTE: Make sure the pressure is fully released before opening the lid, so you do not get burnt.

9. Serve meatloaf topped with fresh cilantro sprigs.

Nutritional info

Calories: 390

Fats (g): 35

Net carbs (g): 8.4

Protein (g): 30

Pot Roast (Italian)

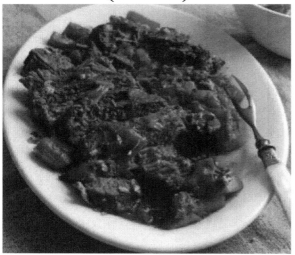

Cook Time: 30 minutes

Servings: 4-6

Ingredients

> 3 pounds beef rump roast, trimmed excess fat and cut into 2" chunks
>
> 1 can/jar sun dried tomatoes in olive oil, chopped
>
> 1 can/jar roasted red bell pepper, julienne sliced
>
> 1 whole onion, thin
>
> 1 can/jar marinated artichokes in water, chopped
>
> 1 mushrooms package, chopped
>
> 1 whole garlic, minced
>
> 2 tablespoons Italian seasoning

Instructions

1. Put 3-4 cups water and meat into Instant Pot, and season with pepper and salt.
2. Close the lid, and turn the vent to "Sealed".
3. Press "Manual" button, set the timer for 10 minutes and set "Pressure" to high.
4. Once the timer is up, press "Cancel" button and allow the pressure to be released naturally, until the float valve drops down.
5. Open the lid.

NOTE: Make sure the pressure is fully released before opening the lid, so you do not get burnt.

6. Take out cooked meat from Instant Pot, and get rid of cooking juices.
7. Rinse cooked roast before putting back into Instant Pot.
8. Add everything else, including liquids and olive oils from artichokes, sun dried tomatoes and bell peppers and do not drain.
9. Put garlic, mushrooms, onions and Italian seasoning into Instant Pot.
10. Close the lid, and turn the vent to "Sealed".
11. Press "Manual" button, set the timer for 20 minutes and set "Pressure" to high.
12. Once the timer is up, press "Cancel" button and allow the pressure to be released naturally, until the float valve drops down. Open the lid.

Nutritional info

Calories: 350

Fats (g): 35

Net carbs (g): 6

Protein (g): 30

Beef Curry Stew

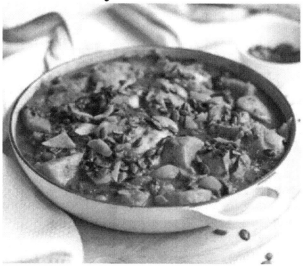

Cook Time: 50 minutes

Servings: 6

Ingredients

2 1/2 pound beef stew chunks, chopped into small cubes

2 zucchinis, chopped

1/2 pound broccoli florets

2 tablespoons curry powder

½ cup water or chicken broth

1 tablespoon garlic power

14 oz can coconut milk

salt, to taste

Instructions

1. Put every ingredient into Instant Pot, and stir until evenly mixed.
2. Close the lid, and turn the vent to "Sealed".
3. Press "Manual" button, set the timer for 45 minutes and set "Pressure" to high.
4. Once the timer is up press "Cancel" button and turn the steam release handle to "Venting" position for quick release, until the float valve drops down.
5. Open the lid.

NOTE: Make sure the pressure is fully released before opening the lid, so you do not get burnt.

6. Add coconut milk and stir with a wooden spoon until evenly mixed.
7. Salt to taste.

Nutritional info

Calories: 180

Fats (g): 25

Net carbs (g): 6

Protein (g): 30

Baby Back Ribs

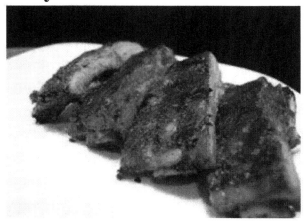

Cooking Time: 50 minutes

Servings: 1 slab of ribs

Ingredients

　　1 meaty slab baby back ribs

　　1/2 cup water

　　2 teaspoons kosher salt

　　1 cup BBQ sauce

　　2 tablespoons BBQ rub

Instructions

1. Remove back ribs membrane.
2. Season baby back ribs with barbecue rub and kosher salt, and cut ribs into four pieces.
3. Pour water into Instant Pot and add seasoned ribs bones side down.
4. Close the lid, and turn the vent to "Sealed".
5. Press "Manual" button, set the timer for 30 minutes.

6. Once the timer is up, press "Cancel" button and allow the pressure to be released naturally, until the float valve drops down.
7. Open the lid.

NOTE: Make sure the pressure is fully released before opening the lid, so you do not get burnt.

8. Top cooked ribs with BBQ sauce and put on a baking sheet.
9. Set "Temperature" to high, cook for 5 minutes (approx) until sauce bubbles and ribs are browned.
10. Top cooked ribs with more BBQ sauce.

Nutritional info

Calories: 360

Fats (g): 35

Net carbs (g): 7

Protein (g): 22

Balsamic Beef Pot Roast

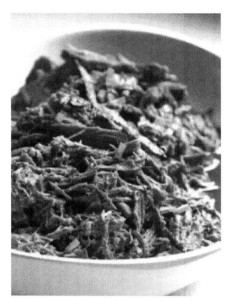

Cooking Time: 45 minutes

Servings: 8 (4 oz)

Ingredients

    1 (3 pounds) boneless chuck roast, cut in half

    1 teaspoon black ground pepper

    1 tablespoon kosher salt

    1/4 cup balsamic vinegar

    1 teaspoon garlic powder

    1/2 cup chopped onion

    2 cups water

    1/4 teaspoon xanthan gum

    fresh parsley, chopped

Instructions

1. Mix garlic powder, pepper and salt, in a mixing bowl.

2. Season a pork roast evenly with the garlic powder mixture.
3. Put seasoned pork roast into Instant Pot.
4. Press "Sauté" button and brown the pork roast for 5-7 minutes both sides with the lid open.
5. Add onion, water and balsamic vinegar into Instant Pot and mix all the ingredients to incorporate.
6. Close the lid, and turn the vent to "Sealed".
7. Press "Manual" button, set the timer for 35 minutes and set "Pressure" to high.
8. Once the timer is up press "Cancel" button and turn the steam release handle to "Venting" position for quick release, until the float valve drops down.
9. Open the lid.

NOTE: Make sure the pressure is fully released before opening the lid, so you do not get burnt.

10. Take meat out and let it cool slightly. Remove any large fat pieces and cut into chunks.
11. Press "Sauté" button on Instant Pot.
12. Bring meat juices to a boil and simmer for 10 minutes until thickened slightly, then add xanthan gum.
13. Add meat chunks and stir until well incorporated.
14. Press "Cancel" button and serve meat over cauliflower rice/puree.
15. Garnish with fresh chopped parsley.

Nutritional info

Calories: 420

Fats (g): 35

Net carbs (g): 6

Protein (g): 23

Faux Cauliflower Mash

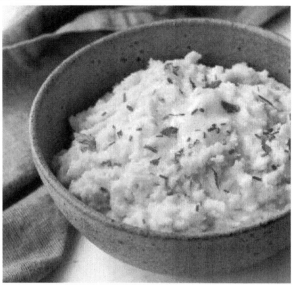

Cooking Time: 5 minutes

Servings: 4 servings

Ingredients

      1 large head cauliflower, cored & cut into large chunks

      1 cup water

      1/8 teaspoon salt

      1 tablespoon butter (if desired)

      1/4 teaspoon garlic powder

      1/8 teaspoon pepper

      1 handful chives (if desired)

Instructions

1. Place a steamer basket or a trivet into Instant Pot.

2. Put cored cauliflower chunks into the steamer basket and add water into the pot.
3. Close the lid and turn the vent to "Sealed".
4. Press "Manual" button, set the timer for 3-5 minutes.
5. Once the timer is up press "Cancel" button and turn the steam release handle to "Venting" position for quick release, until the float valve drops down.
6. Open the lid and carefully put water out of Instant Pot.

NOTE: Make sure the pressure is fully released before opening the lid, so you do not get burnt.

7. Put softened cauliflower back into Instant Pot and add salt, garlic powder, pepper; butter and chives (if desired).
8. Puree the mixture with an immersion blender until it is of a desired consistency.

Nutritional info

Calories: 62

Fats (g): 6

Net carbs (g): 4.8

Protein (g): 3

Brussels Sprout Recipe

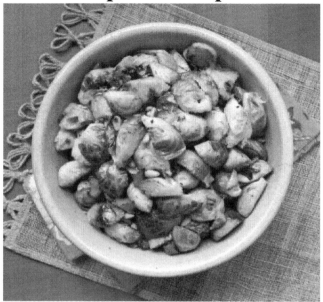

Cooking Time: 3 minutes

Servings: 2-4 servings

Ingredients

    1 pound Brussels sprouts
    salt, to taste
    1 cup water
    olive oil
    1/4 cup pine nuts
    pepper, to taste

Instructions

1. Place a steamer basket into Instant Pot.

2. Add water and put Brussels sprouts into the steamer basket.
3. Close the lid and turn the vent to "Sealed".
4. Press "Manual" button, set the timer for 3 minutes and set "Pressure" to high.
5. Once the timer is up press "Cancel" button and turn the steam release handle to "Venting" position for quick release, until the float valve drops down.
6. Open the lid.

NOTE: Make sure the pressure is fully released before opening the lid, so you do not get burnt.

7. Add pepper, salt and olive oil to Brussels sprouts.
8. Top with sprinkled pine nuts.

Nutritional info

Calories: 197

Fats (g): 25

Net carbs (g): 3.1

Protein (g): 10

Spaghetti Squash

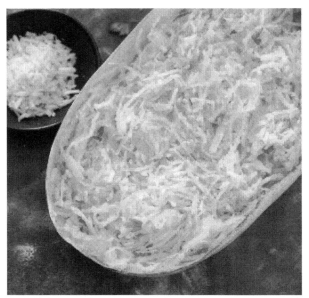

Cooking Time: 10 minutes

Servings: 2 servings

Ingredients

    1 cup water

    1 medium spaghetti squash, cut in half crosswise, seeds removed

Instructions

1. Place a steamer basket into Instant Pot.
2. Add water and put the spaghetti squash into the steamer basket with cut side up.
3. Close the lid and turn the vent to "Sealed".

4. Press "Manual" button, set the timer for 7 minutes and set "Pressure" to high. For a softer squash cook for 1-3 minutes longer.

5. Once the timer is up press "Cancel" button and turn the steam release handle to "Venting" position for quick release, until the float valve drops down.

6. Open the lid.

7. NOTE: Make sure the pressure is fully released before opening the lid, so you do not get burnt.

8. Shred spaghetti squash with a fork and add your desired keto topping or sauce.

Nutritional info

Calories: 51

Fats (g): 9

Net carbs (g): 5

Protein (g): 18

Steamed Artichokes

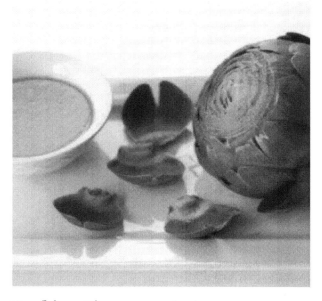

Cooking Time: 30 minutes

Servings: 2-4 servings

Ingredients

  1 lemon wedge

  2 (5 1/2 oz. each) medium-sized whole artichokes, rinsed, stem & top third removed

  1 cup water

Instructions

1. Use a lemon wedge to rub every cut top of the artichokes to stop browning.
2. Place a steamer basket or a steam rack into Instant Pot.
3. Put the artichokes into the steamer basket and add water.
4. Close the lid and turn the vent to "Sealed".

5. Press "Manual" button, set the timer for 20 minutes and set "Pressure" to high.
6. Once the timer is up, press "Cancel" button and allow pressure to be released naturally, until the float valve drops down.
7. Open the lid.

NOTE: Make sure the pressure is fully released before opening the lid, so you do not get burnt.

8. Carefully take the artichokes out with tongs and serve with desired dipping sauce.

Nutritional info

Calories: 31

Fats (g): 11

Net carbs (g): 6.9

Protein (g): 15.1

Cauliflower Soup & Creamed Fennel

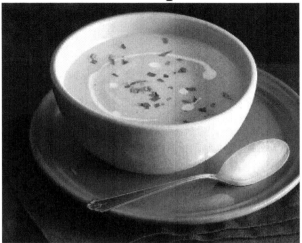

Cooking Time: 30 minutes

Servings: 4 servings

Ingredients

    1 tbsp coconut oil

    3 garlic cloves, minced

    1 white onion, sliced

    1 lb. cauliflower florets

    2 medium sized fennel bulbs, fronds and stalks removed, then chopped

    3 cups vegetable or bone broth

    1 cup coconut milk

    2 teaspoons salt

For Serving:

    black pepper and Truffle oil

Instructions

1. Put coconut oil to Instant Pot and press "Sauté" button.
2. Put onions and cook until soft and translucent with the lid open.
3. Add cauliflower, fennel and garlic and keep cooking for 5 to 10 minutes until the vegetables edges start to become golden.
4. Press "Cancel" button, pour coconut milk and broth into Instant Pot.
5. Close the lid and turn the vent to "Sealed".
6. Press "Soup" button and set timer for 7 minutes.

7. Once the timer is up press "Cancel" button and turn the steam release handle to "Venting" position for quick release, until the float valve drops down.
8. Open the lid.

NOTE: Make sure the pressure is fully released before opening the lid, so you do not get burnt.

9. Puree soup to creamy and smooth consistency with an immersion blender.
10. Serve in bowls, spring some truffle oil.
11. Top with pepper and garnish with a fennel frond that was left over. Enjoy while hot.

Nutritional info

Calories: 220

Fats (g): 35

Net carbs (g): 7

Protein (g): 20

Cream Sauce Savoy Cabbage

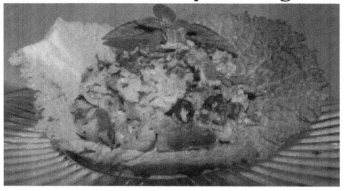

Cooking Time: 9 minutes

Servings: 4-6 servings

Ingredients

    1 cup diced lardon or bacon

    2 cups bone broth

    1 onion, chopped

    ¼ teaspoon nutmeg or mace

    1 (approx. 2 pounds) finely chopped, medium Savoy cabbage head

    1 bay leaf

    ½ can (approx. 1 cup) coconut milk

    2 tablespoons parsley flakes

    sea salt, as needed

Instructions

1. Cut parchment paper to fit the inner and put aside.

2. Press "Sauté" button. Put onion and bacon into Instant Pot, cook until onion is translucent and slightly browned, and the bacon is crispy.
3. Add bone broth and scrape with wooden spoon to loosen browned bits.
4. Add bay leaf and cabbage into Instant Pot and stir until incorporated.
5. Place the parchment paper on the top to cover the dish.
6. Close the lid, and turn the vent to "Sealed".

7. Press "Manual" button, set the timer for 4 minutes and set "Pressure" to high.
8. Once the timer is up press "Cancel" button and turn the steam release handle to "Venting" position for quick release, until the float valve drops down.
9. Open the lid.

NOTE: Make sure the pressure is fully released before opening the lid, so you do not get burnt.

10. Remove the parchment paper and press "Sauté" button.
11. Add coconut milk and nutmeg or mace into Instant Pot.
12. Cook for 5 minutes with the lid open, then press "Cancel" button.
13. Stir in parsley flakes until combined.

Nutritional info

Calories: 180

Fats (g): 25

Net carbs (g): 4

Protein (g): 10

Bacon & Collard Greens

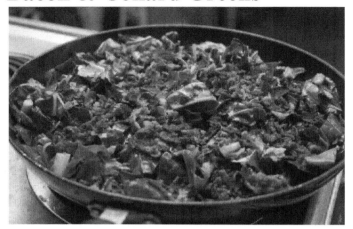

Cooking Time: 30 minutes

Servings: 6-8 servings

Ingredients

> 1/4 lb. bacon, cubed or sliced into small strips
>
> 1/2 tsp kosher salt
>
> 1 lb. collard greens, stems trimmed, chopped
>
> black pepper, to taste
>
> 1/2 cup water

Instructions

1. Put bacon into Instant Pot.
2. Press "Sauté" button, cook for 5 minutes with the lid open, and stir bacon from time to time until crispy and browned.
3. Add half of collards and stir until wilted a little.
4. Add another half of collards and stir until fully wilted.

NOTE: Collards wilt very fast so there will be enough space for other ingredients in your Instant Pot.

5. Add salt and water, close the lid and turn the vent to "Sealed".
6. Press "Manual" button, set the timer for 20 minutes and set "Pressure" to high.
7. Once the timer is up press "Cancel" button and turn the steam release handle to "Venting" position for quick release, until the float valve drops down.
8. Open the lid.

NOTE: Make sure the pressure is fully released before opening the lid, so you do not get burnt.

9. Season with black pepper.

Nutritional info

Calories: 200

Fats (g): 30

Net carbs (g): 5

Protein (g): 15

Elegant Shrimp Dish

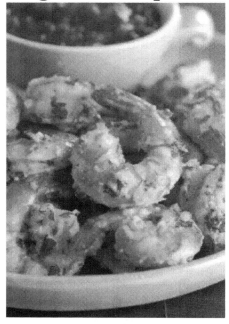

Cooking time: 5 minutes

Servings: 4

Ingredients

    2 tablespoons parsley, chopped

    1 cup yellow onion, chopped

    1 and ½ pounds shrimp, peeled and deveined

    2 tablespoon olive oil

    ½ cup fish stock

    2 teaspoons hot paprika

    4 garlic cloves, minced

    ¼ cup white wine

    1 cup tomato sauce

    A pinch of saffron

½ teaspoon sugar

1 bay leaf

¼ teaspoon thyme, dried

1 teaspoon hot red pepper, crushed

a pinch of pink salt

black pepper, to taste

Instructions

1. Put oil into Instant Pot, press "Sauté" button and heat it up.
2. Add shrimp, stir, cook for 1 minute with the lid open, transfer to a bowl and leave aside for now.
3. Add onion, stir and sauté it for 2 minutes.
4. Add wine, garlic, paprika and parsley, stir and cook for 2 minutes.
5. Add saffron, sugar, stock, tomato, red pepper, bay leaf, thyme, salt and pepper, stir and close the lid, set the timer for 4 minutes and set "Pressure" to high.
6. Once the timer is up press "Cancel" button and turn the steam release handle to "Venting" position for quick release, until the float valve drops down.
7. Add shrimps, close the lid again, set the timer for 4 minutes and set "Pressure" to high.
8. Repeat step 6.

Nutritional info

Calories: 385

Fats (g): 14.7

Net carbs (g): 6.1

Protein (g): 34.3

Paella

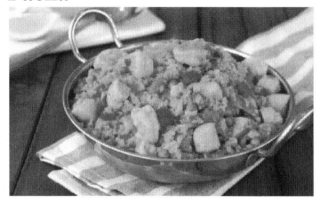

Cooking time: 5 minutes

Servings: 4

Ingredients

    1 cup cauliflower rice

    20 big shrimp, deveined

    a pinch of red pepper, crushed

    ¼ cup parsley, chopped

    a pinch of sea salt

    black pepper, to taste

    ¼ cup ghee

    a pinch of saffron

    1 and ½ cups water

    juice from 1 lemon

    4 garlic cloves, minced

    cheddar cheese, grated

Instructions

1. Add water to Instant Pot.
2. Press "Sauté" button, put rice.

3. Add shrimps, ghee, parsley, salt, pepper, red pepper, lemon juice, saffron, garlic and water, stir for 1-2 minutes with the lid open.

4. Close the lid, and turn the vent to "Sealed".
5. Press "Manual" button, set the timer for 5 minutes and set "Pressure" to high.
6. Once the timer is up press "Cancel" button and turn the steam release handle to "Venting" position for quick release, until the float valve drops down.
7. Open the lid.

NOTE: Make sure the pressure is fully released before opening the lid, so you do not get burnt.

8. Peel shrimps and divide them on plates.
9. Add rice mix on top, parsley and grated cheese.

Nutritional info

Calories: 151

Fats (g): 11.4

Net carbs (g): 5.8

Protein (g): 7.1

Shrimp and Sausages

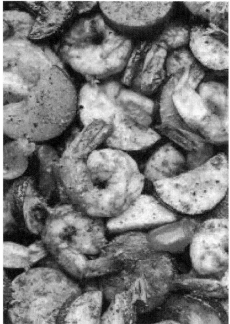

Cooking time: 5 minutes

Servings: 4

Ingredients

12 oz sausage, cooked and sliced
1 and ½ pounds shrimp, deveined
1 tablespoon old bay seasoning
1 zucchini, thinly sliced
16 oz beer
a pinch of sea salt
black pepper, to taste
2 yellow onions, cut in wedges
1 teaspoon red pepper flakes, crushed

8 garlic cloves, minced

Instructions

1. Put beer, old bay seasoning, pepper flakes, salt, pepper, garlic, onions, sausage, zucchini and shrimp into Instant Pot and stir.
2. Close the lid.
3. Press "Manual" button, set the timer for 5 minutes and set "Pressure" to high.
4. Once the timer is up press "Cancel" button and turn the steam release handle to "Venting" position for quick release, until the float valve drops down.
5. Open the lid.

NOTE: Make sure the pressure is fully released before opening the lid, so you do not get burnt.

6. Divide into bowls and serve.

Nutritional info

Calories: 210

Fats (g): 25

Net carbs (g): 8

Protein (g): 16

Shrimp Curry

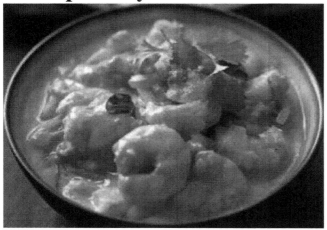

Cooking time: 30 minutes

Servings: 4

Ingredients

> 1 cinnamon stick
>
> 2 bay leaves
>
> 1 pound shrimp, deveined and peeled
>
> 1/3 cup butter
>
> 2 red onions chopped
>
> 10 cloves
>
> 3 cardamom pods
>
> 14 red chilies, dried and crushed
>
> ½ cup cashews
>
> 1 tablespoon garlic paste
>
> 3 green chilies, chopped
>
> 1 tablespoon ginger paste
>
> a pinch of sea salt
>
> 1 teaspoon sugar

4 tomatoes, chopped

1 teaspoon fenugreek leaves, dried and crushed

½ cup cream

Instructions

1. Put butter into Instant Pot, press "Sauté" button and heat it up.
2. Add cardamom, cinnamon stick, bay leaves and onion, stir and cook for 3 minutes with the lid open.
3. Add green chilies, cashews, garlic paste, cloves, ginger paste, red chilies and a pinch of salt, stir.
4. Close the lid, set the timer for 15 minutes and set "Pressure" to high.
5. Once the timer is up press "Cancel" button and turn the steam release handle to "Venting" position for quick release, until the float valve drops down.

NOTE: Make sure the pressure is fully released before opening the lid, so you do not get burnt.

6. Pour this mix into your food processor and blend well.
7. Return this into Instant Pot, add shrimp, stir a bit.
8. Close the lid, Press "Manual" button, set the timer for 8 minutes and set "Pressure" to high.
9. Once the timer is up release pressure, open the lid, add cream, sugar and fenugreek.
10. Press "Simmer" button, stir and simmer for 5 minutes.

Nutritional info

Calories: 230

Fats (g): 25

Net carbs (g): 5

Protein (g): 10

Salmon Burger

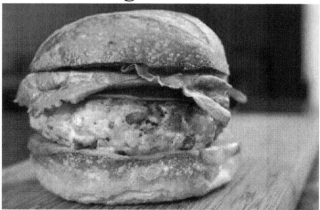

Cooking time: 10 minutes

Servings: 4

Ingredients

    1 pound salmon, ground

    2 tablespoons lemon zest

    black pepper to taste

    a pinch of salt

    1 teaspoon olive oil

    ½ cup panko

    For serving:

    mustard

    tomato slices

    arugula leaves

Instructions

1. Blend salmon with panko, salt, pepper and lemon zest in your food processor.

2. Stir the mix well, shape 4 burger patties and place them on a plate.
3. Press "Sauté" button, add oil and heat Instant Pot up, put patties there.
4. Close the lid, set the timer for 10 minutes and set "Pressure" to high.
5. Once the timer is up, press "Cancel" button and allow the pressure to be released naturally, until the float valve drops down.

NOTE: Make sure the pressure is fully released before opening the lid, so you do not get burnt.

6. Open the lid.
7. Press "Sauté" button again and cook patties for 2 minutes more.
8. Divide salmon patties on buns, add tomato slices, arugula and mustard.

Nutritional info

Calories: 460

Fats (g): 40

Net carbs (g): 8

Protein (g): 25

White Fish

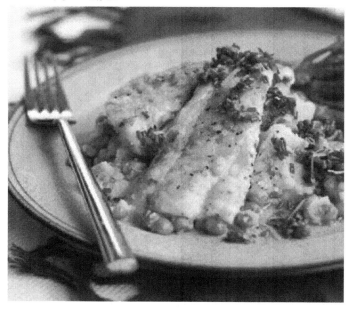

Cooking time: 25 minutes

Servings: 6

Ingredients

  1 yellow onion, chopped
  6 white fish fillets, cut in chunks
  salt and black pepper, to taste
  1 cauliflower head, separated into florets
  13 oz milk
  14 oz chicken stock
  14 oz half and half
  14 oz water

Instructions

1. Put cauliflower florets, fish, onion, milk, stock and water into Instant Pot, stir everything.
2. Close the lid, press "Manual" button, set the timer for 10 minutes and set "Pressure" to high.
3. Once the timer is up press "Cancel" button and turn the steam release handle to "Venting" position for quick release, until the float valve drops down.
4. Open the lid.
5. Press "Simmer" button, add half and half, salt and pepper, stir and cook for 10 minutes more.

Nutritional info

Calories: 270

Fats (g): 35

Net carbs (g): 4

Protein (g): 15

Salmon with Special Raspberry Sauce

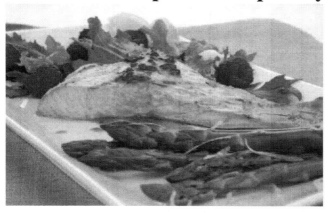

Cooking time: 5 minutes

Servings: 6

Ingredients

    4 leeks, chopped

    2 tablespoons olive oil

    6 salmon steaks

    2 garlic cloves, minced

    1 cup clam juice

    2 tablespoons parsley, chopped

    2 tablespoons lemon juice

    1/3 cup dill, chopped

    1 teaspoon sherry

    a pinch of sea salt

    black pepper, to taste

    2 pints red raspberries

    1 pint cider vinegar

Instructions
1. Mix raspberries and vinegar in a bowl and stir well.
2. Add salmon, stir, cover and keep in the fridge for 2 hours.
3. Put oil into Instant Pot and press "Sauté" button.
4. Add garlic, parsley and leeks, stir and cook for 2 minutes with the lid open.
5. Add lemon juice, clam juice, salt, pepper, cherry and dill, stir and cook for 2 minutes.
6. Add salmon steaks, stir.
7. Close the lid, set the timer for 4 minutes and set "Pressure" to high.
8. Once the timer is up, press "Cancel" button and allow the pressure to be released naturally, until the float valve drops down.

NOTE: Make sure the pressure is fully released before opening the lid, so you do not get burnt.

9. Serve hot.

Nutritional info
Calories: 160

Fats (g): 25

Net carbs (g): 5

Protein (g): 12

Cauliflower Fritters

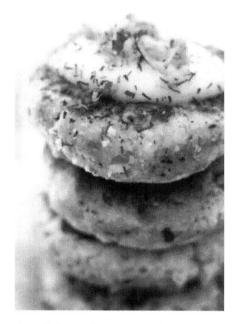

Cooking time: 6 minutes

Servings: 5

Ingredients

  1 head cauliflower, cut into florets

  2 tablespoons olive oil

  salt, to taste

  ½ cup almond meal

  2 eggs

  2 tablespoons all-purpose flour

  2 tablespoons Greek yogurt

  1 garlic clove, grated

  1½ teaspoon curry powder

1 teaspoon cumin powder

½ teaspoon turmeric powder

¼ teaspoon cinnamon powder

handful cilantro, chopped

1 tablespoon oil

Instructions

1. Season cauliflower with salt, drizzle some oil on it.
2. Place a steamer basket or a trivet into Instant Pot.
3. Put cauliflower into the steamer basket and add water into the pot.
4. Close the lid and turn the vent to "Sealed". Press "Manual" button, set the timer for 3-5 minutes.
5. Once the timer is up press "Cancel" button and turn the steam release handle to "Venting" position for quick release, until the float valve drops down.
6. Let cauliflower cool and blend it a bit in food processor.
7. Transfer the cauliflower into a bowl and mix with almond meal, eggs, flour, yogurt, spices and salt.
8. Chill for a couple of hours and then make small patties.
9. Press "Sauté" button, add oil and heat Instant Pot up, put patties there.
10. Close the lid, set the timer for 10 minutes.
11. Once the timer is up, press "Cancel" button and allow the pressure to be released naturally, until the float valve drops down.

NOTE: Make sure the pressure is fully released before opening the lid, so you do not get burnt.

12. Open the lid.
13. Put fritters on a paper towel and serve hot.

Nutritional info

Calories: 170

Fats (g): 15

Net carbs (g): 5

Protein (g): 10

Bacon Poppers

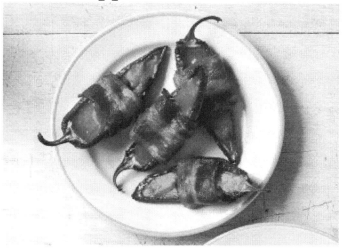

Cooking time: 5 minutes

Servings: 5

Ingredients

    1 tablespoon oil

    12 Jalapeño peppers, halved and deseeded

    1 cup ricotta cheese

    ½ cup Gruyère cheese, grated

    12 slices bacon, cut lengthwise

    2 tablespoons fresh cilantro, chopped

    1 cup water

Instructions

1. Mix cheeses with cilantro until evenly combined.
2. Fill jalapeño halves with this mixture.

NOTE: Use gloves when slicing and filling peppers if you do not want your fingers to burn.

3. Add oil to Instant Pot, press "Sauté" button. Put bacon, cook until slightly browned.
4. Take bacon out and pour water into Instant Pot.
5. Wrap each jalapeño halve with bacon slices and place them on a trivet.
6. Close the lid, press "Manual", set the timer for 5 minutes and set "Pressure" to high.
7. Once the timer is up, press "Cancel" button and allow the pressure to be released naturally, until the float valve drops down.

NOTE: Make sure the pressure is fully released before opening the lid, so you do not get burnt.

Nutritional info

Calories: 434

Fats (g): 13.5

Net carbs (g): 3.5

Protein (g): 24.2

Cauliflower Tots

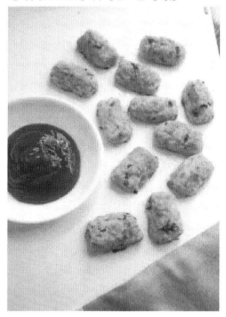

Cooking time: 5 minutes

Servings: 50

Ingredients

1 medium cauliflower head, cut into florets

2 tablespoons heavy cream

2 tablespoons butter

1 cup water

1/3 cup sharp cheddar cheese, shredded

4 egg whites

salt and black pepper, to taste

Instructions

1. Add cream and butter to cauliflower florets.
2. Place a steamer basket or a trivet into Instant Pot.
3. Put cauliflower into the steamer basket and add water into the pot.
4. Close the lid and turn the vent to "Sealed". Press "Manual" button, set the timer for 3-5 minutes.
5. Once the timer is up press "Cancel" button and turn the steam release handle to "Venting" position for quick release, until the float valve drops down.
6. Allow cauliflower cool to room temperature.
7. Blend it with food processor or immersion blender.
8. Season it with salt and black pepper.
9. Chill this mixture for an hour.
10. Meanwhile, whip egg whites. Add egg whites into cauliflower mixture until combined. Chill again.
11. Add oil to Instant Pot, form small cauliflower nuggets and put them there.
12. Press "Saute" button, add oil and heat Instant Pot up, put patties there.
13. Close the lid, set the timer for 10 minutes and set "Pressure" to high.
14. Once the timer is up, press "Cancel" button and allow the pressure to be released naturally, until the float valve drops down.
15. Open the lid.

Nutritional info

Calories: 864

Fats (g): 63

Net carbs (g): 18

Protein (g): 47

Split Asparagus Soup Recipe

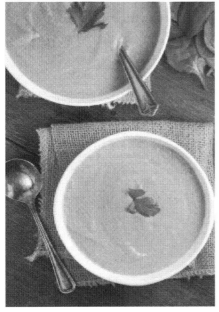

Cooking Time: 30 minutes

Servings: 4-6 servings

Ingredients

   2 pounds asparagus, chopped in half

   5 garlic cloves, pressed

   3 tablespoons ghee

   1 cup diced ham or 1 ham bone

   1 white onion, diced

   1/2 teaspoon thyme, dried

   4 cup chicken broth

   pepper, to taste

   salt, to taste

Instructions

1. Put ghee into Instant Pot, press "Sauté" button, melt it.
2. Add diced onion into melted ghee and cook until the onion is brown for approximately 5 minutes, with the lid open.
3. Add broth, ham bone and pressed garlic.
4. Sauté for 2-3 minutes, then add asparagus and thyme.
5. Close the lid, and turn the vent to "Sealed".
6. Press "Soup" and set the timer for 45 minutes.

7. Once the timer is up, press "Cancel" button and allow the pressure to be released naturally, until the float valve drops down.
8. Open the lid.

NOTE: Make sure the pressure is fully released before opening the lid, so you do not get burnt.

9. Blend soup with a food processor or immersion blender.

Nutritional info

Calories: 220

Fats (g): 45

Net carbs (g): 5

Protein (g): 23

Kale & Chicken Soup

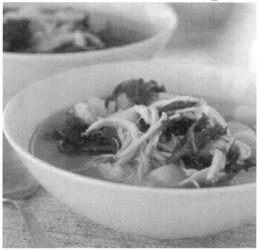

Cooking Time: 9 minutes

Servings: 4 servings

Ingredients

2 tablespoons olive oil or butter

3 carrots, peeled & cut into small bite-sized pieces

1 medium onion, chopped

2 bay leaves

4 celery stalks, cut into small bite-sized pieces

1/2 teaspoon black pepper

1 teaspoon salt

1/4 teaspoon oregano, dried

1/2 teaspoon thyme, dried

1 pound chicken breast, cooked, shredded

4 cups chicken broth + 1 cup water

1/2 teaspoon Worcestershire sauce or fish sauce

1 cup kale, chopped

Instructions

1. Put butter or oil into Instant Pot.
2. Press "Sauté" and add onions.
3. Sauté for 5 minutes with the lid open, until soft.
4. Add oregano, thyme, pepper, salt, bay leaves, celery and carrots into Instant Pot.
5. Keep sautéing for 1 more minute, until fragrant.
6. Add water and broth into Instant Pot.
7. Close the lid and turn the vent to "Sealed".
8. Press "Soup", set the timer for 4 minutes and set "Pressure" to high.
9. Once the timer is up press "Cancel" button and turn the steam release handle to "Venting" position for quick release, until the float valve drops down.
10. Open the lid.

NOTE: Make sure the pressure is fully released before opening the lid, so you do not get burnt.

11. Add kale and chicken into Instant Pot and let sit for 1 minute until kale turns bright green.
12. Add pepper, salt and fish sauce and stir to incorporate.

Nutritional info

Calories: 240

Fats (g): 29

Net carbs (g): 4

Protein (g): 14

Cauliflower Soup

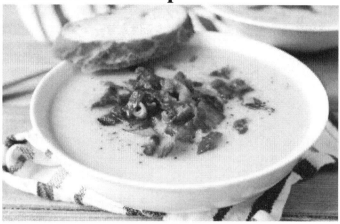

Cooking Time: 10 minutes

Servings: 4-6 small servings

Ingredients

    1/2 small onion, peeled & chopped

    1 large cauliflower head, steam, leaves and chop removed

    2 tablespoons olive oil or butter

    1 teaspoon garlic powder

    3 cups (24 oz) homemade chicken stock

    4 oz cream cheese, cubed

    1 teaspoon kosher salt

    1/2 cup milk or half and half

    1 cup grated cheddar cheese

For serving:

    cheddar cheese, grated

    8-10 bacon strips, cooked crisp & crumbled

sour cream

green onions, thin-sliced

Instructions

1. Put butter or oil into Instant Pot.
2. Press "Sauté" button, add onions and sauté for 2-3 minutes with the lid open.
3. Add salt, garlic powder, chicken stock and chopped cauliflower into Instant Pot.
4. Close the lid and turn the vent to "Sealed".
5. Press "Manual", set the timer for 5 minutes and set "Pressure" on high.

6. Once the timer is up press "Cancel" button and turn the steam release handle to "Venting" position for quick release, until the float valve drops down.
7. Open the lid, make sure cauliflower is well cooked and soft.

8. NOTE: Make sure the pressure is fully released before opening the lid, so you do not get burnt.
9. Press "Keep warm" and blend soup with an immersion blender until of a desired consistency.

NOTE: Be careful as cauliflower soup will be hot. Add more chicken stock to thin soup if necessary.

10. Add cream cheese cubes and grated cheese into soup and stir until melted.
11. Put half and half into Instant Pot and warm up slightly.
12. Add pepper and salt and check for seasoning, adding more pepper and salt to taste.
13. Serve hot, topped with sliced green onions, crumbled bacon, sour cream, and grated cheese.

Nutritional info

Calories: 320

Fats (g): 45

Net carbs (g): 10

Protein (g): 27

Chili Lime Steak Bowl Recipe

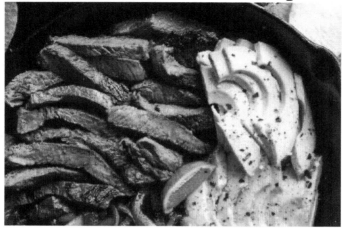

Cooking Time: 15 minutes

Servings: 4 servings

Ingredients

      1.2-2 lbs. beef steak strips

      1 garlic clove, minced

      1 tablespoon water

      2 teaspoons lime juice

      1 tablespoon EVOO

      1/2 teaspoon sea salt

      1/2 teaspoon chili powder

      1 teaspoon Cholula

      1/2 teaspoon cracked pepper

      2-3 avocado, diced

Instructions

1. Add olive oil into Instant Pot.
2. Press "Sauté" button, add garlic and sauté until browned.
3. Add water, lime juice, sea salt, chili powder, Cholula, cracked pepper and stir with a wooden spatula.
4. Close the lid and turn the vent to "Sealed".
5. Press "Manual" button, set the timer for 10 minutes and set "Pressure" on high.
6. Once the timer is up press "Cancel" button and turn the steam release handle to "Venting" position for quick release, until the float valve drops down.
7. Open the lid.

NOTE: Make sure the pressure is fully released before opening the lid, so you do not get burnt.

8. Press "Sauté" button, add steak strips and stir with a wooden spoon for couple of minutes.
9. Continue sautéing until chili becomes thicker and reduced by 1/2.
10. Serve with diced avocados.

Nutritional info

Calories: 250

Fats (g): 35

Net carbs (g): 3

Protein (g): 15

Beef Soup

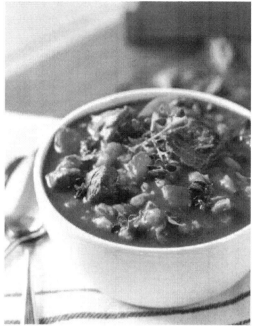

Cooking Time: 25 minutes

Servings: 3-4 servings

Ingredients

    2 lbs. beef stew meat
    1 onion, sliced
    2 tablespoons cooking oil
    4 garlic cloves
    4 carrots, peeled & sliced
    1 cup water
    3 cups beef broth
    2 bay leaves
    1 tablespoon tomato paste

6 thyme sprigs

Instructions

1. Season meat with salt and pepper.
2. Press "Sauté" button, add oil and stir meat until browned, for 3-5 minutes.
3. Add garlic, carrots and onions into and brown for few minutes.
4. Add thyme sprigs, bay leaves, tomato paste and broth into Instant Pot and stir to combine.
5. Close the lid and turn the vent to "Sealed".
6. Press "Manual" button, set the timer for 30 minutes and set "Pressure" to high.
7. Once the timer is up, press "Cancel" button and allow the pressure to be released naturally, until the float valve drops down.
8. Open the lid.

NOTE: Make sure the pressure is fully released before opening the lid, so you do not get burnt.

9. Check for seasoning, add pepper and salt to taste.

Nutritional info

Calories: 330

Fats (g): 65

Net carbs (g): 3

Protein (g): 25

71350500R00066

Made in the USA
Lexington, KY
20 November 2017